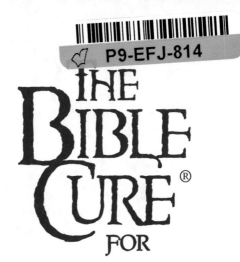

THE BIBLE CURE® FOR

ALLERGIES

DON COLBERT, M.D.

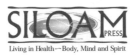

Living in Health—Body, Mind and Spirit

THE BIBLE CURE FOR ALLERGIES
by Don Colbert, M.D.
Published by Siloam Press
A part of Strang Communications Company
600 Rinehart Road
Lake Mary, Florida 32746
www.creationhouse.com

Unless otherwise noted, all Scripture quotations
are from the Holy Bible, New Living Translation,
copyright © 1996, Tyndale House Publishers,
Inc., Wheaton, Illinois 60189.

Scripture quotations marked KJV are from the
King James Version of the Bible.

Library of Congress Catalog Card Number:
99-85848

International Standard Book Number:
0-88419-685-2

0 1 2 3 4 5 6 VERSA 8 7 6 5 4 3 2
Printed in the United States of America

Preface

You *Will*
Feel Better!

God desires that you feel better, healthier—and even younger! Stop sneezing and wheezing from allergies that drain you, drag you down and rob you of energy and joy! God's wonderful Word says:

> Praise the LORD, I tell myself, and never forget the good things he does for me. He forgives all my sins and heals all my diseases. He ransoms me from death and surrounds me with love and tender mercies. He fills my life with good things. My youth is renewed like the eagle's!
> —PSALM 103:2–5

This powerful Bible verse reveals how much

God loves you and desires for you to feel really good. If you battle constant or seasonal wars against allergies, you're not alone. Statistics show that more than a third of the entire American population suffers alongside of you.

One-Third of All Americans Sneeze, Drain, Drip and Cough

Allergies affect about 38 percent of all Americans—almost twice as many as allergy experts once believed. According to a new survey released by the American College of Allergy, Asthma and Immunology, millions rely on medications unnecessarily because they don't know about other effective treatment options.[1]

Allergic reactions are not God's plan for you. God's mighty Word promises, "'For I know the plans I have for you,' says the LORD. 'They are plans for good and not for disaster, to give you a future and a hope. In those days when you pray, I will listen. If you look for me in earnest, you will find me when you seek me. I will be found by you'" (Jer. 29:11–14).

Be Encouraged and Energized!

As you read this booklet, you will discover ways to

avoid those things that cause allergies in your life. You will also begin to feel better physically, emotionally and spiritually. This Bible Cure booklet is filled with practical steps, hope, encouragement and valuable information on how to stay fit and healthy. In this book, you will

> *uncover God's divine plan of health*
> *for body, soul and spirit*
> *through modern medicine, good nutrition*
> *and the medicinal power*
> *of Scripture and prayer.*

You will discover life-changing healing scriptures throughout this booklet that will strengthen and energize you.

As you read, apply and trust God's promises, you will also uncover powerful Bible Cure prayers to help you line up your thoughts and feelings with God's plan of divine health for you—a plan that includes living victoriously. In this Bible Cure booklet, you will be equipped to overcome your allergies in the following chapters:

There is much you can do to overcome allergies and defeat the miserable symptoms that accompany them. This Bible Cure plan will energize you with confidence, determination and knowledge to live allergy free! God's healing power is greater than any allergy attack you may now be facing.

A Bold, New Strategy

This Bible Cure booklet is dynamically packed with powerful natural and spiritual solutions to combat and defeat your allergy symptoms. This booklet will examine allergy-producing agents and provide ways to eliminate and combat them. You will also uncover healthy ways to eat and a powerful strategy for taking vitamins and supplements that will strengthen your immune system and reduce your allergy symptoms. God will help you discern those agents that are causing your allergic reactions, and He will give you the knowledge, understanding and determination to take the necessary steps to live allergy free.

So, don't be discouraged. Your Bible Cure for allergies is in God's plan for your life. He desires for you to walk in divine health free from the misery of allergy symptoms. God's desire for you is found in 3 John 2, "Dear friend, I am praying that all is well with you and that your body is as healthy as I know your soul is."

I believe that the power of faith in God's wonderful Word and the divine touch of His healing hand, together with the practical suggestions for allergy-free living outlined in this book, will restore your breath, health, energy, vitality and joy!

—DON COLBERT, M.D.

A BIBLE CURE PRAYER
FOR YOU

I pray that the almighty God, who is our Savior and our Healer, will give you wisdom and discernment as you read this book. I pray that all that will help you in these pages will be made relevant to you and easy to remember. I pray that all you learn will cause you to live allergy free. Amen.

Chapter 1

All About Allergies

When God created mankind, He placed us in a beautiful environment that was perfectly suited for us. The Bible says, "Then God looked over all he had made, and he saw that it was excellent in every way" (Gen. 1:31).

God declared that all of creation was "excellent," meaning it was wholesome, pure, healthy and beneficial. Nothing in it would harm the human body—it was a perfect environment. However, humankind polluted God's wonderful creation. Today's world is poisoned with toxins in the air we breathe, in the water we drink and in the food we eat.

If you have allergies, you may already be well aware of the allergens in the world around you and their impact upon your body. But don't be discouraged. Your coughing, wheezing, running nose, watery eyes and other symptoms can be stopped naturally by taking positive steps to remove toxins from your environment and to control what you eat.

As you read this booklet you may discover some surprises about yourself, especially if you are suffering from less understood allergy symptoms such as depression, panic attacks, mental confusion and insomnia.

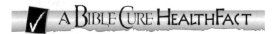
A BIBLE CURE HEALTHFACT

The most common allergies are:

- Allergic rhinitis (hay fever), with symptoms that include nasal stuffiness, sneezing, nasal itching, clear nasal discharge and itching of the roof of the mouth and/or ears
- Allergic asthma, with symptoms of wheezing, coughing and shortness of breath
- Allergic conjunctivitis (an eye allergy), which produces redness, itching and a chronic mucus-related discharge
- Allergic eczema, which is an allergic skin rash

- Allergic contact dermatitis, e.g., poison ivy
- Food allergies

What Is Causing Your Allergies?

Allergies are a result of a breakdown of our immune systems. For you see, God has created an incredible immune system for each and every one of us. It has been designed to identify and differen-

> *And it is a good thing to receive wealth from God and the good health to enjoy it. To enjoy your work and accept your lot in life—that is indeed a gift from God.*
> —ECCLESIASTES 5:19

tiate between what our bodies actually need and what is alien or foreign to them. When our immune systems encounter foreign products, they produce antibodies, which cause white blood cells to release histamines. This in turn causes the symptoms of watery, itchy eyes and nose, sneezing, drainage and so forth. A foreign substance may be bacteria, a virus or a parasite. The wonderful immune system vigilantly protects against these foreign invaders.

However, problems arise when foods, animal

hair, dust, mold and pollens stimulate an antibody's response, causing an inflammatory reaction. This inflammatory reaction can affect different organs and eventually lead to fatigue and degenerative diseases.

Driving Your Ferrari

An allergic person's immune system is similar to driving a high-powered Ferrari sports car with weak brakes. When attempting to stop at high speeds, your weak brakes can cause the vehicle (the immune system) to spin out of control. This loss of immune system control leads to recurring infections such as sinusitis, bronchitis, ear infections and arthritis. All of these illnesses cause the immune system to work continually so that it eventually weakens even more. When an individual's immune system begins to break down, he or she then becomes susceptible to all kinds of diseases.

Imagine that a food designed to nourish the body could actually rev up the immune system instead. When this happens, the GI tract can become inflamed, which may lead to food allergies. The allergic reaction cycle spirals at increasing rates, which eventually leads to chronic degenerative diseases.

A Full Tank

We might picture the immune system as a gas tank. Our energy level will be high if we keep our tank full (or strong) by improving our nutrition, cleaning up our environments and taking vitamins and supplements.

Keeping our immune systems strong gives our bodies the power to fight physical attacks, so we can resist most allergic reactions and diseases. However, if our tanks become empty, or if our immune system reserves become depleted, then any excess stress—such as is produced by inadequate sleep, exposure to fumes or cigarette smoke and excessive stress at work—will impact us. When our immune systems become weakened, the strength of allergic reactions can overcome the body's ability to resist them. When this occurs, we begin sneezing and coughing, our noses run and our eyes get itchy. Allergy symptoms come into full bloom.

Let's look at some natural methods to keep your tank full or to strengthen your immune system.

Taking a Closer Look

There are five types of allergic reactions that an individual may experience.

Type one

Type one reactions are the reactions you may have to animal dander, pollen, dust, mold and so on. An immediate hypersensitivity reaction occurs, usually within two hours. When the body comes into contact with these materials, it releases histamine and other by-products.

The allergy symptoms that follow depend upon from where the body's cells release the histamine. If the cells release their allergy-producing substances in the nasal passages, then sneezing, runny nose and congestion may occur. If the bronchial tubes are involved, then wheezing may occur. If the site is the skin, then eczema or hives may occur.

Type one reactions account for only about 10 to 15 percent of all food allergy reactions. This means that only 1 to 2 percent of all adults are allergic to foods or experience a "type one immediate hypersensitivity reaction." Since type one reactions occur in such a small percentage of those who suffer from allergies, it is easy to see why doctors often overlook food allergy symptoms.

Type two

Type two reactions occur when an allergic substance unites with a healthy cell, and then antibodies (large proteins that fight off foreign invaders such as bacteria and toxins) actually destroy the good cell. This often occurs in the cells of the intestines and leads to diarrhea, bloating and indigestion, nausea, abdominal cramps, spastic colon, belching and flatulence.

Type three

Type three reactions are caused when allergy-producing substances attach to antibodies to destroy them and form a substance called an "immune complex." These complexes can then be deposited into certain tissues of the body and, as a result, injure the tissues.

Type four

Type four reactions occur, for example, when an individual gets poison ivy. When special cells (called T-cells) become stimulated at a particular location on the body, such as the skin, a type four allergic reaction takes place. The stimulated cells create an inflammation at the particular site, such as the skin, the lungs or the GI tract.

Food-hypersensitivity reactions

Some allergic reactions to food are not even triggered by the immune system. These are known as food-hypersensitivity reactions. They occur when no allergen antibody response is present, but an adverse reaction to food still takes place. For simplicity's sake, I will be referring to food sensitivities or hypersensitivities as food allergies, too.

Take this little quiz to help you better understand how allergies work.

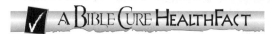

Allergy Quiz

1. Allergies always start during childhood. (True or False)

False—Although many people experience the onset of allergies when they are children, allergies can begin at any age. Adult-onset allergies are becoming increasingly common. The symptoms are the result of an abnormal sensitivity of the immune system to particular allergens—substances that are usually harmless. Allergies can also flare up and subside throughout an individual's lifetime.

2. Allergies that make you sneeze and sniffle usually go away after the first frost because below-freezing temperatures kill most allergens. (True or False)

False—Even though frost kills pollen-producing plants such as grasses, weeds and ragweed, other allergens such as molds, dust mites and animal dander persist year round.

3. The best way to avoid allergies caused by airborne pollen is to stay indoors. (True or False)

False—Avoiding allergens is the first line of defense for those who suffer from allergies, but there are other ways you can minimize contact with these allergens without staying indoors all the time. A critical step is knowing what to avoid. An allergist, a doctor who specializes in allergies, can help you to identify the things that trigger your allergic responses and can then help you develop an avoidance program that will work for you.[1]

HEALTHFACT HEALTHFACT HEALTHFACT HEALTHFACT HEALTHFACT HEALTHFACT HEALTHFACT

I believe that we are surrounded by more allergens today than at any other time in history. Thousands of new products and new chemicals are being developed year after year, which often find their way into our food, water and air. So over time we will eventually be exposed to many of these chemicals. Also, much of what we eat contains flavorings, preservatives, food additives and stabilizers that can cause food allergies as well.

Food Allergies

Food allergies are certainly not new. More than two thousand years ago Hippocrates, who was a Greek physician known as the father of medicine, described food allergies when he noted that cheese caused severe reactions in some men while others could eat it without any reaction whatsoever.

Allergies can also be caused by foods, beverages and any product that is ingested—even vitamin supplements. Most food allergy symptoms are delayed from a couple of hours to a couple of days, whereas inhalant allergen symptoms are usually immediate—that is, within a couple of hours. Substances that come in contact with your skin can also cause allergic reactions.

A Leaky Gut

A common cause of food allergies is a syndrome known as "leaky gut syndrome." A leaky gut is simply a damaged lining of the small intestines. The cells of this lining become flattened and inflamed. When this occurs, nutrients cannot be properly absorbed by the body, which leads to food allergies.

A leaky gut is exactly what it sounds like. Holes in the mucous membrane of the GI tract, caused by injury, infection or anything else, allow molecules of food to move directly into the bloodstream. These molecules then cause allergic responses that take place in the intestinal walls, creating symptoms such as diarrhea, nausea, bloating, belching and gas.

This condition is also associated with bacterial overgrowth in the small intestines, stress, candidiasis, parasitic infections and the use of alcohol and anti-inflammatory medications such as Advil, Motrin, Nuprin and store brands of ibuprofen.

When an individual is experiencing a leaky gut, foods are absorbed through the intestines more easily. The intestines normally function to absorb materials that are beneficial to the body and to act as a barrier to materials that can harm the body.

A leaky gut allows whole food proteins such as albumin from eggs, casein from milk, gluten from wheat and other proteins from other foods to be absorbed directly into the circulatory system. Antibodies are then formed against these proteins. When these foods are eaten again, the antibodies signal that a toxic invader has entered the system, and inflammatory reactions begin to occur in the GI tract. In other words, the lining of the GI tract becomes the battlefield where antigens (which is the allergic food) and antibodies meet. Food that should be nourishing our bodies actually begins to

11

drain our immune systems by stimulating inflammatory reactions in the intestinal walls.

In addition, candida yeast can actually attach itself to the walls of the GI tract and form rootlike structures and damage the lining of the GI tract. These rootlike structures are called *mycelia*. They thus cause inflammation of the intestines as well as leaky gut.

What Causes Food Allergies?

The most common foods that cause allergies include eggs, milk products and wheat. Other allergens include chemicals, such as hydrocarbons, pesticides, industrial chemicals and solvents. They can also include medicines or vaccines that have been injected, including PPD, injections for TB, childhood immunizations and injectible medications. Allergens also may include chemicals that come in contact with the skin such as poison ivy, cosmetics, hair dyes, nail polish, formaldehyde, gasoline, latex gloves, animal dander (or fur) and detergents. Also, emotional stress while eating can stimulate food allergies.

Food Allergy Symptoms

Food allergies are associated with many different

medical conditions that can impact almost every part of the body. Symptoms of food allergies include sore throats, recurrent sinus infections, sneezing, postnasal drip, hoarseness, earaches, ringing in the ears, recurrent ear infections and itching in the ears.

Respiratory symptoms caused by food allergies may include cough, asthma, bronchitis and wheezing.

Intestinal tract symptoms may include diarrhea, indigestion, gas, spastic colon, nausea, abdominal cramps, constipation, increased belching, increased flatulence, indigestion and acid stomach.

Skin symptoms may include hives, eczema, psoriasis, dark circles under the eyes, itching and acne.

Your nervous system can also be affected by allergies. Symptoms may include:

- Depression
- Weakness
- Panic
- Hyperactivity
- Poor memory
- Insomnia
- Hallucinations
- Fatigue
- Anxiety
- Confusion
- Decreased concentration
- Delusions
- Nightmares

Urinary symptoms may include frequency of urination, an urgency to urinate, bedwetting and pain during urination.

Muscular and skeletal problems may include muscle aches and pains, muscle weakness, muscle stiffness, stiff joints, arthritis and low back pain.

Other symptoms may include exhaustion, rapid heartbeats, irregular heartbeats and palpitations. Allergic reactions to foods typically begin within minutes to a few hours after eating the offending food.

In summary, here's a quick checklist of symptoms for food allergies:

- A runny nose with sneezing
- Upper airway swelling of the tongue, lips and throat
- Skin rashes, including hives and eczema
- Intestinal symptoms like vomiting, nausea, stomach cramps, indigestion and diarrhea
- Coughing or wheezing
- Rhinitis, often including itchy, stuffy, runny nose and sneezing
- Anaphylaxis, a severe allergic reaction that may be life-threatening

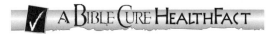

Who Has Food Allergies?

While an estimated forty to fifty million Americans have allergies, only 1 to 2 percent of all adults are allergic to foods or food additives. Eight percent of children under age six have adverse reactions to ingested foods; only 2 to 5 percent have confirmed food allergies.[2]

HEALTHFACT HEALTHFACT HEALTHFACT HEALTHFACT HEALTHFACT HEALTHFACT HEALTHFACT

Environmental Allergies

While much legislation has been passed to help clean up our air and water, we continue to face a number of irritating toxins that trigger allergic reactions.

Many environmental factors can cause allergies. I'd like to focus on the broadest category: inhalants. Inhalants are materials you inhale or breathe into your body. They include any of the following materials (check the inhalants that you suspect may be causing your allergy symptoms):

❑ Pollen, such as tree weed and grass pollens
❑ Mold spores

- ❏ Dust
- ❏ Dust mites
- ❏ Animal dander
- ❏ Smoke
- ❏ Chlorine gas
- ❏ Perfumes
- ❏ Cosmetics
- ❏ Chemical fumes
- ❏ Paint
- ❏ Cooking aromas

Inhalant allergy symptoms

The symptoms of inhalant allergies include sneezing, runny nose, sore throats, recurrent sinus infections, hoarseness and itchy, watery, red eyes. A telltale sign of inhalant allergies is allergic shiners, or dark circles under the eyes. Another sign is the "allergic salute," or the upward swiping motion of the palm of the hand to the nose, which creates a horizontal crease across the nose.

Get Ready to Feel Better!

Allergies are often complicated problems, and discovering their causes can be complicated as well. It is possible to be allergic to more than one food or environmental factor—and those factors can change throughout your lifetime and even throughout the seasons of a year. It may take some prayer, determination and effort, but you can and will discover the causes of your allergies and begin to work on the solutions.

Even if you don't immediately understand your allergies entirely, the Bible Cure steps you will find in the remaining chapters of this little book will prove very helpful. By strengthening your body, correcting a few environmental factors and learning to draw greater emotional and spiritual strength from God, you will soon discover that you feel much better—physically, mentally and emotionally!

A BIBLE CURE PRAYER
FOR YOU

Almighty God, Creator of the universe, I give You praise for Your good and glorious creation. Thank You for creating clean air and water. Reveal to me the causes of allergic reactions in my body. Give me the discernment and wisdom to understand what I am eating or inhaling that is causing an allergic reaction in my body. I thank You that You desire for me to walk in divine health. Amen.

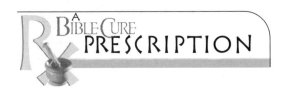

A BIBLE CURE PRESCRIPTION

Describe any symptoms you have for the following:

Common food allergies

1. Eggs _____

_____

2. Dairy _____

_____

3. Wheat products _____

_____

Common inhalant allergies

1. Dust _____

_____

2. Pollen (trees, weeds, grass) _____

_____

3. Mold _____

_____

4. Animal dander (cats, dogs, birds) _____

_____

5. Smoke _____

_____

List any habits you have that may produce allergic reactions:

_____

_____

_____

_____

_____

Describe what you have learned about allergies:

_____

_____

_____

_____

_____

Chapter 2

Attacking Allergies
Through Nutrition

The ancient writer Lucretius said, "What is food for one is to others bitter poison." When an individual responds to a commonly harmless food as through he were poisoned, he is displaying a food allergy.

God has created an abundance of natural foods for us to eat. Genesis 1:29–30 reveals, "And God said, 'Look! I have given you the seed-bearing plants throughout the earth and all the fruit trees for your food. And I have given all the grasses and other green plants to the animals and birds for their food.'"

God created the foods our bodies need for nourishment and growth. But each individual's body does not respond to those foods in the same way.

You may be experiencing allergies to certain foods because of heredity, because of the toxins contained in those foods when they are processed, due to an injured GI tract from drinking alcohol or taking aspirin, anti-inflammatory medications, antibiotics or yeast. This chapter will help you identify the foods you may be allergic to and give you positive steps for eliminating those foods from your diet.

Take It Slow:
Eight Nutritional Tips

Let's see, you're not even sure what you're allergic to—if anything. You can still prevent many allergic reactions long before they begin, or reverse them once they've started, by taking some simple nutritional steps. Here are eight important ways to take it a little slower, live a lot longer and enjoy the ride a little more as you go. If you have children, these eight steps can create a foundation for starting them out in life with nutritional habits that will help them to build allergy-free futures.

1. Be slow to introduce solids.
Don't give your infant solid foods too soon. Starting your infant on solid foods too early can cause food allergies, especially if your baby isn't

breastfed. The best way to prevent food allergies in children is to breastfeed them as infants for the first six months of life before starting solids.

2. Be slow to chew and swallow.

Chew your food well. Did you know that poor digestion is closely linked to food allergies? Poor digestion starts with chewing food improperly. This, together with inadequate hydrochloric acid and pancreatic enzymes (digestive acids), will lead to incomplete digestion, which can cause a leaky gut.

3. Avoid aspirin.

Avoid aspirin, alcohol, ibuprofen, antibiotics and environmental toxins. Yeast overgrowth in the small intestines and bacterial overgrowth caused by the items listed above may damage the immune barrier and create leaky gut syndrome.

4. Limit liquids.

Don't drink more than four ounces of fluid during a meal. It's even better to drink your beverage thirty minutes before a meal. Many individuals drink large amounts of fluids with their meals and wash down their food with a beverage instead of chewing it thoroughly. Too much liquid while eating can dilute pancreatic enzymes. Therefore, limit fluids during meals.

5. *Add enzymes.*

Some individuals may actually need to supplement their meals with enzymes, and some actually need hydrochloric acid. Get a comprehensive physical exam by a nutritional doctor and have a comprehensive digestive stool analysis to check for pathogenic bacteria, overgrowth of yeast or parasites.

6. *Get good bacteria.*

Take in good bacteria—which includes lactobacillus acidophilus and bifidus—to re-colonize the GI tract. You can replenish your body with good bacteria by eating plain yogurt.

7. *Introduce interesting foods.*

Don't eat the same foods all the time. Food allergies are also caused by excessive and repeated consumption of the same foods, especially for a person with leaky gut syndrome.

8. *Watch out for chemicals in foods.*

Finally, I believe that more and more individuals are experiencing food allergies because of the excessive chemical pollutants that we are consuming in our food and water. Make an extra effort to select foods and liquids based upon purity and freshness. Avoid processed foods that contain a lot of chemicals, and check out the organic vegetable section at your grocers. Organic foods are grown free of toxic chemicals and additives and are much better for you.

These simple, basic measures can help your intestines to absorb only well-digested nutrients into your blood stream, which is a giant first step in preventing food allergies.

A Lineup of Suspects

Your offending foods are probably among the lineup of usual suspects listed below. The most common food allergens include eggs, milk products, wheat, yeast, corn, sugar and soy. Get a good look at them and see if you can identify any of their symptoms so that you can avoid them in your diet.

The problem with proteins

Any food can cause an allergic reaction. However, high-protein foods tend to be the greatest offenders. You see, proteins are much more difficult to digest than carbohydrates or even fats. If proteins pass into the bloodstream before they are digested, the protein molecules that are absorbed into the bloodstream remain too large. Therefore, the immune system then recognizes the large protein molecules as foreign invaders instead of nutrients. It then launches an effort to destroy the invader.

Limit meats

Meats cause allergies much more often than fruits and vegetables. Grains also frequently cause allergies, especially the grains that contain gluten, such as wheat, oats, rye and barley. Cooking foods decreases this effect by about half. Eating organic foods also decreases the allergic effect, because most commercially prepared meats are contaminated with pesticides, antibiotics and growth hormones, all of which can cause allergies. Cooking foods in oils, such as olive oil, slows the absorption rate of the food during digestion and therefore decreases allergic reactions.

✓ A BIBLE CURE HEALTHFACT

Here is a list of painful and sometimes embarrassing physical reactions that are linked to what you eat.

- Asthma can be triggered by milk, eggs, chocolate, nuts, peanuts, seafood and corn, as well as other foods.

- Colitis and Crohn's disease can be associated with allergies to milk, tomatoes, eggs, wheat, corn and nuts, as well as other foods.

- Ear infections are commonly related to milk allergy. However, eggs, corn and wheat may also be involved, as well as other foods.

- Arthritis is commonly associated with nightshades including tomatoes, potatoes, eggplant, bell peppers, chili peppers and pimientos. Other foods that can trigger joint inflammation include pork, wheat and sugar, as well as other foods.

- Bedwetting is commonly triggered by milk, chocolate, corn, wheat and eggs, as well as other foods.

- Eczema is commonly associated with a milk allergy. It also may be due to chocolate, eggs, grains and beans, as well as other foods.

- Hyperactivity may be caused by food additives and may also be due to corn, sugar and wheat allergies, as well as other foods.

- Migraine headaches can be triggered by milk, eggs, wheat, chocolate, wine, nuts, pork or corn, as well as other foods.

Avoid eggs

Eggs contain the protein albumin, which is a substance that many individuals are allergic to. If you are allergic to eggs, avoid cakes, candies, cookies, desserts, ice cream, mayonnaise, pancakes, pasta, pastries, puddings, salad dressings, waffles, pretzels and doughnuts. Processed foods offer little nutritional value, and even those of us who are not allergic to eggs are better off avoiding them.

Never eat raw eggs! They are often contaminated with the bacteria salmonella. Do you like your eggs lightly cooked, such as sunny side up, soft poached or lightly scrambled? You still can run a higher risk of developing salmonella. Why not try cooking your eggs a little longer?

Eggs also contain pesticide residue, antibiotics and other drugs. Therefore, I choose organic varieties. The taste is the same or better, and the health risks are drastically reduced.

Limit milk

Milk is a very common food allergen because

of the protein casein. Lactalbumin is another protein found in milk that may cause bloating, gas and diarrhea in many people. Lactose is found in milk sugar and in cream and causes allergic reactions in many other milk drinkers. It may surprise you to know that the following products all contain milk: cakes, all cheeses, cookies, candy bars, hot dogs, ice cream, pancakes, salad dressings, waffles, yogurt and butter.

Symptoms of milk allergies may include asthma, rashes, nasal congestion, ear infections, diarrhea and hyperactive behavior. Patients with Crohn's disease should also be tested for milk allergy.

It's easy to get the calcium your body needs from sources other than milk and milk products. These sources include soybeans, broccoli, almonds, fish and different kinds of beans, including pinto beans and kidney beans.

Reduce wheat

Wheat is a common allergen in the United States. It contains more of the protein gluten than any other grain. Rye, barley and oats contain lesser amounts of this protein, and corn, rice and millet contain none at all.

Gluten is also present in many processed foods. Some of the most common foods that contain wheat are bread, buns, cakes, candy, cereals, hamburger mix, chocolate, cookies, macaroni, pizza, bologna, mayonnaise, monosodium glutamate (MSG), pasta, pancakes, pretzels and crackers.

Evade yeast

Do you love that wonderful yeasty smell from freshly baked bread? If you are allergic to yeast, you must avoid eating it. Yeast is commonly used in baked goods and also in alcoholic beverages. Yeast converts sugar to alcohol and carbon dioxide. Foods that contain yeast include barbecue sauce, breads, cakes, ketchup, cheese, coffee, cookies, crackers, nuts, all alcoholic beverages, flour, fruit juices, cantaloupe, mushrooms, peanuts, pizza, pretzels, rolls, sour cream, soy sauce, vinegar, mayonnaise, mustard, pickles, salad dressings, tomato sauce and olives.

Refuse sugar

Do you crave sugar? Sugar is another common food allergen. The average adult consumes about 150 pounds of it a year.[1] Sugar is rapidly absorbed into our bodies, and it can cause severe reactions in those who are allergic to it. It can also be quite addictive. Sugar depletes the body of B vitamins as well as chromium, magnesium and manganese. Sugar stresses both our adrenal glands and pancreas.

Common sugars include the following:

- Corn sweeteners are used in most baked goods, ice cream, ham, bacon, sausage, ketchup and soft drinks.
- Sucrose is cane sugar and comes from both sugar cane and sugar beets. This is used in ice cream, jellies, jams and processed meats.
- Dextrose is a derivative of cornstarch and is used in intravenous solutions.
- High-fructose corn syrup is produced from dextrose and is an ingredient in all soft drinks. It is also used in cereals, salad dressings, ketchup and baked goods.
- Glucose is also derived from cornstarch. It is not nearly as sweet as sucrose and is found in luncheon meats and ham.
- Fructose is twice as sweet as sucrose and is found in cakes, candies, jellies, cereals, mayonnaise and salad dressings.
- Honey is 80 percent sucrose but requires

31

no digestion by humans. Often corn syrup
or other sugars are added to honey.

Cut out corn

Corn is used in so many different foods that it
is probably the most difficult allergen to eliminate
from the diet. Corn-containing products include
all carbonated beverages, breads, cakes, candies,
ketchup, cereals, crackers, fruit juices, ham,
liquor, beer, pies, salad dressings, tacos, tortillas
and vinegar. The list goes on and on. It is even
used in toothpaste.

Shun soy

Soy is also a common allergen in the U.S. Soy
beans have been grown in the U.S. for approximately two hundred years, and more and more
uses for soy are being created. However, this is one
of the most allergic foods we can have in our diets.
Common sources of soy include baked goods,
candies, cereals, ice cream, meats, pasta, salad
dressings, margarine and sauces, including soy
sauce, teriyaki sauce and Worcestershire sauce.

Exactly What Are You Allergic To?

Now that you've examined a lineup of the usual

offenders, you may be wondering exactly which ones are personally offending you. Allergies are as individualistic as eye color and height. Attacking food allergies in your own life will require determining exactly which foods are attacking you.

The simplest way to treat food allergies is to avoid any food you may be allergic to. But first you must identify the food allergen. Several testing methods listed below can help you. In addition, an elimination diet and journal are provided at the end of this book that will help you to understand exactly what foods are causing your allergy symptoms. Begin creating your own allergy profile by asking yourself what foods, if any, you crave.

> *If you will listen carefully to the voice of the LORD your God and do what is right in his sight, obeying his commands and laws, then I will not make you suffer the diseases I sent on the Egyptians; for I am the LORD who heals you.*
> —EXODUS 15:26

What Are You Craving?

One of the nurses in my practice is allergic to sugar. Every time she eats a dessert or other high-sugar food for lunch, she becomes increasingly sleepy, spacey and forgetful by midafternoon. Her ability to work is dramatically affected by simply having a piece of pie or cake. She is allergic to the very foods she craves.

Do you crave certain foods? Food cravings are a telltale sign that you are allergic to those foods. Does that seem impossible to you? It's not. In addition to craving the very foods that are making you ill, if you have a food allergy you probably even feel better after eating the offending foods. If you try to stop eating what you allergic to, you may discover that you experience withdrawal symptoms.

This is the reason that so many food allergies go undetected and untreated. You may not cough, sneeze or experience nasal congestion, but a food allergy can make you feel sleepy or give you a headache an hour or so after you've eaten.

Your pulse rate is another good indicator of food allergies.

Getting a Pulse on Your Food Allergies!

You can usually determine if you are allergic to a food by simply monitoring your pulse rate. Record your pulse rate both before and after eating a particular food. Take your pulse for one minute, and then eat the food. Take your pulse again five minutes after eating. Follow up by taking your pulse at fifteen-minute intervals for the following hour.

If your pulse rate increases over ten beats per minute after eating a particular food, then there is a very strong possibility that you may be allergic or sensitive to that food.

An even simpler way to do this is to take your pulse for one minute before eating a food that you suspect you are allergic to and then putting the food on your tongue for thirty seconds. Retest your pulse for one minute. If your pulse rate increases more than ten beats, you are probably allergic to that food, and you will then be able to avoid it in the future.

Allergy tests administered by physicians are very accurate. Let's look at a few of them.

Allergy Tests Your Doctor Can Give You

Lab tests can be performed to determine if you have food allergies. The ALCAT assesses the size and number of an individual's white blood cells both before and after he or she is exposed to food allergens. The RAST (Radioallergosorbent Test) measures the level of antibodies found in the blood after an individual has been exposed to a food or allergen. The ELISA (Enzyme-Linked Immunosorbent Assay) test measures many different antibodies that play a major role in food allergies.

Allergy tests using fasting methods are also very effective. Let's examine some of these.

Test for Allergies by Fasting

A simple way to find out which foods you are allergic to is to fast for four to five days and then reintroduce foods one at a time. After the four- to five-day elimination period, test the foods that are suspect by eating only one food item at a time and then monitoring your reactions over the next three to four hours after consuming the food. Add only one food per day, and record any reactions immediately after eating and again several hours after eating.

Once you have identified your allergens, whether they are wheat, eggs, milk, corn, yeast, sugar or soy, then avoid eating any of those allergens for four days. It takes the body that long to clear the food that you have eaten. By rotating the diet you reduce allergic reactions by preventing the buildup of antibodies to these foods.

Meal Replacements and
Hypoallergenic Diets

As an alternative to fasting, you may use a hypo-allergenic meal replacement formula such as UltraInflamX from Health Designs or Ultraclear from Metagenics. (You can find these products through the Internet at www.healthdesigns.com or www.metagenics.com respectively.) Or, you may eat a hypoallergenic diet, which includes eating all fruits (except for citrus, berries and tomatoes), all nonstarchy vegetables, turkey, whitefish such as halibut and sole, almonds, sunflower seeds and white or brown rice. If you've tested positive to a particular food, then avoid it for three months if you are highly allergic. Rotate foods you are mildly or moderately sensitive to every four days. If you eat any foods regularly or crave them, rotate them every four days also; do not eat them daily. Refer to page 71 for the Elimination Diet that I commonly use in my practice.

It has been my experience, however, that most people will not follow this diet unless they are highly motivated. Therefore, I use this method only for the most severely allergic individuals who have exhausted other options.

Fasting and special allergenic diets are usually a last resort. If you are an average allergy sufferer, you can probably discover all you need to know by less rigorous methods, especially if you have an understanding of your family's allergy history.

Your Family Tree

Did your mother break out in hives after she ate tomatoes? Did your father get sleepy after eating a Sunday dinner of pot roast and gravy? Knowing what foods your parents or grandparents were allergic to can provide a clearer understanding of your own symptoms. Genetics play an important part when it comes to food allergies, so take time to gather information about your genetic pre-disposition to allergies.

You Are Not
an Allergy Victim!

Understanding your own genetic factors can give you important insight into your symptoms and those of your children as well. However, you are not a victim of genetics, your environment or any-thing else. If you believe in God's power to heal, you are never merely a statistic, for you have already beaten all the odds. Faith in God is a principle that transcends the mathematics of any actuarial table, graph or chart!

Wisdom From Above

Do you lack understanding of what foods are causing your allergy symptoms? Ask God. He promises to answer you. The Bible says, "If you need wisdom—if you want to know what God wants you to do—ask him, and he will gladly tell you. He will not resent your asking. But when you ask him, be sure that you really expect him to answer" (James 1:5–6).

Ask God to reveal to you what foods are causing your allergy symptoms, and then begin taking the Bible Cure steps I've just outlined. As you look to God for answers, expect to find great relief. God loves you dearly and cares deeply about everything in your life. You will discover, as I have, that having faith in God will never disappoint you.

A BIBLE CURE PRAYER
FOR YOU

Lord, help me to discover the foods I am allergic to and to eliminate them from my diet. Right now I cast all my cares on You, knowing that You care for me. Help me to avoid foods that are not good for me. Give me the desire to eat healthy so that my body will be a strong vessel for serving You. Amen.

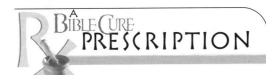

A BIBLE CURE PRESCRIPTION

List the foods you know you are allergic to:

_____

_____

_____

_____

Describe what you are doing to avoid a leaky gut:

_____

_____

_____

What foods do you need to eliminate from your diet?

_____

_____

_____

Chapter 3

Attacking Allergies Through Environment

God is the mighty Creator who shaped the earth as a dazzling reflection of His own glory and majesty. The Bible says, "O LORD God Almighty! Where is there anyone as mighty as you, LORD? . . . The heavens are yours, and the earth is yours; everything in the world is yours—you created it all" (Ps. 89:8, 11).

The perfection of God's creation must have been truly awesome to behold. Much of it retains the glory of its original splendor. But sadly, mankind has done much to mar that beauty as well. Throughout history, we have filled crystal-clear springs with murky pollutants and yellow, foamy detergents. We have filled our dazzling clear skies with the brownish haze of smog and our rich, loamy soil with toxic chemicals and poisons.

God created pure water, air and food for us. But we have poured a multitude of chemicals into them, especially through automobile exhaust and factory pollution. In its original state, the earth would have never harmed us. However, the accumulation of hundreds of years of pollution, toxins and poisons is taking a heavy toll. And those of us with allergies are paying it!

Allergy sufferers are often at war with their own hostile environments. But there is hope. The same God who created this wonderful earth to strengthen and support you is still as alive, active and powerful as He was on creation morning. He will give you the wisdom you need to adjust your environment so that you can enjoy your life to the fullest extent.

Here are some steps you can take to help you stop sneezing, draining, coughing and wheezing. When you discover the causes for your environmental allergies, address the problem immediately. Take the steps recommended below to modify your environment, and expect to begin feeling better fast.

Take It Away:
Five Environmental Tips

Allergies caused by materials in the air that you

breathe into your lungs, or inhalant allergies, are linked to pollens from trees, weeds and grasses, mold, dust and animal dander. Most of these inhalant allergies cannot be completely avoided, so it's important to make some environmental changes to control them.

1. Take away plant allergens.

Pollen allergies to trees, grasses and weeds occur at different seasons of the year. Some news services actually announce local mold and pollen counts to aid allergy sufferers. If you suffer from pollen allergies, no one needs to tell you that your eyes water and itch and your sinuses drain uncontrollably when pollen counts are up. Your symptoms are worse on windy days and improve when you're indoors or on rainy days.

You can control airborne pollen by using a home air purifier, such as Hepa filters. Ionizers, which use electrical current to cleanse and purify odors and allergies in the air, can help you create a pollen-free environment in the home as well.

2. Take away mold.

Inhalant mold allergies usually do not cause the eyes and nose to itch. But they often cause nasal congestion and chronic sinus problems.

This is because the mold colonizes within the sinuses and nasal passages.

Mold allergy symptoms get worse in cool evening air, in damp places and especially when leaves are being raked. Sufferers also feel worse in damp weather and when they are mowing grass.

If you have mold allergies, you usually will feel better inside of a house, especially when an air conditioner or heating furnace is on. Your symptoms will also decrease when outside temperatures drop below freezing.

A Bible Cure Health Tip

Take these steps to control mold allergies:

- Prevent dampness inside your house.
- Increase air circulation with an air purifying system.
- If the humidity is high in the house, get a dehumidifier.
- Ventilate bathrooms well and use tile flooring in the bathrooms, not carpet.
- Don't keep damp clothing in the bathroom. Take it to the laundry room and hang it up to dry to avoid mildew, which is also caused by mold.

- Discard any bedroom items that have molded, especially foam pillows, bedding, old newspapers and magazines.
- Mold can also thrive in the foam rubber padding underneath your carpet. If you have mold allergies, it's best to have tile or hardwood floors in your bedroom.
- Decorative plants should also be removed from the house since they harbor mold.
- Keep all firewood out of the house since mold grows on the bark of the trees.
- Clean shower walls and floors with bleach, since this kills mold.
- Make sure to dry any standing water in the bathroom.
- Air purifiers, ionizers and ozone generators will also remove mold spores. However, the filters must be changed periodically.

3. Take away animal dander.

Do you wheeze and sneeze around cats? Animal dander (fur), especially cat dander, is an extremely strong allergen for humans. Have you ever noticed how often and how thoroughly a cat will lick its coat? Cat saliva is extremely allergenic.

Dog dander is another common cause of allergies, but it is not as allergenic as cat dander.

Symptoms of allergies to cats or dogs include wheezing, itchy, watery eyes, sneezing, hives and hoarseness. Don't get rid of your cat too quickly, though. You can drastically reduce your allergy symptoms by regularly bathing your pet.

4. *Take away dust.*

Household dust contains both organic and inorganic dirt. It is comprised of mold spores, pollen, cellulose lint from cotton, linen and other fibers, animal dander and minute bits of cockroaches, silverfish, spiders, fleas, flies, dust mites, insect feces and human dander. The average six-room house will accumulate approximately forty pounds of dust in a year.

Dust allergy symptoms will usually worsen after you have been vacuuming or dusting the house or when you make your bed. Symptoms will generally be more severe when you first get up in the morning, and they will improve throughout the day. If you are allergic to dust, you will usually feel worse indoors and better when you go outside.

It's impossible to avoid dust completely, but you can control it significantly. Start in your bedroom.

Don't store items under your bed that will act as dust collectors. Wash all your blankets and bedspreads at least once a month. If your bedroom is carpeted, have the carpet removed. Replace it with tile or hardwood flooring. In addition, remove drapes and blinds; use curtains that can be washed instead.

Remove dust catchers such as pictures, bric-a-brac, artificial flowers and the like. Keep all pets out of the bedroom, and keep closet doors closed at all times. Cover mattresses and pillows. Vacuum and dust your bedroom floor and furniture every day. Get a room air purifier and change the filter regularly.

If your children are allergic to dust, don't fill their rooms with stuffed toys. Finally, try to avoid going into attics, storage rooms or any other dust-filled areas.

> *Don't worry about anything; instead, pray about everything. Tell God what you need, and thank him for all he has done. If you do this, you will experience God's peace, which is far more wonderful than the human mind can understand. His peace will guard your hearts and minds as you live in Christ Jesus.*
> —PHILIPPIANS 4:6–7

5. Take away dust mites.

Dust mites live in dust and are relatives of ticks and spiders. They survive on the millions of skin scales shed by people every day. Each dust mite produces about twenty fecal pellets a day—pellets so light that they actually float in the air for as long as ten minutes. These dust mites usually live in mattresses, furniture, stuffed animals and carpets.

If you are allergic to dust mites, your symptoms include nasal congestion, stuffiness of the ears and a lot of sneezing, especially upon rising out of bed. Your symptoms improve when you are outdoors but worsen when you make your bed.

The best way to control dust mites is to control the humidity in your house with a dehumidifier. Using central heating will also decrease your home's dust mite population significantly. Mattress and pillow covers are helpful, too.

✓ A BIBLE CURE HEALTHFACT

Our more sedentary lifestyles, brought about by televisions, home computers and other forms of home entertainment, may be exposing us to more indoor allergens.

"The consequence of sitting for three or more

hours per day in front of a television, video or computer are decreased activity, increased obesity and increased exposure to indoor allergens," said Dr. Platts-Mills. "Prolonged sitting may also influence lung mechanics and predispose children to asthma."[1]

Additional lifestyle factors that increase allergic reactions are:

- Closed ventilation systems on public transportation, including airplanes
- Decreased ventilation and increased use of carpeting in homes

Ask Your Doctor

Lab tests can be performed to determine if you have environmental allergies. These lab tests include the scratch or prick test, which can diagnose inhalant allergens such as pollens, dust, mold and animal dander. In addition, ask your doctor about a RAST test, which measures the level of antibodies found in the blood after an individual has been exposed to an allergen.

Your doctor knows how important it is to listen to your body's signals, for your body and good health are precious gifts.

Your Body—God's Gift

God created your body to thrive in a healthy environment. Allergy symptoms are a signal that your body is struggling to cope with environmental pollutants that were never God's design. Make every effort to maintain a healthy environment to protect your body and your immune system.

Your body is a unique gift from God. The psalmist wrote:

> You made all the delicate, inner parts of my body and knit me together in my mother's womb. Thank you for making me so wonderfully complex! Your workmanship is marvelous—and how well I know it. You watched me as I was being formed in utter seclusion, as I was woven together in the dark of the womb. You saw me before I was born. Every day of my life was recorded in your book. Every moment was laid out before a single day had passed. How precious are your thoughts about me, O God! They are innumerable!
>
> —Psalm 139:13–17

Since your body is such a precious gift from God, determine to protect it every way possible.

A BIBLE CURE PRAYER
FOR YOU

Lord, thank You for the precious gift of my body and my good health. Help me to protect this body that You have given me from environmental toxins and allergens. Keep me aware of the places I go and the air I breathe. Give me wisdom to keep my home as clean and toxin free as possible. Thank You for this knowledge that makes me aware of how to eliminate allergens and live an allergy-free lifestyle. Amen.

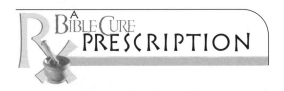

A BIBLE CURE PRESCRIPTION

Check all the things you need to address that might be causing your allergic reactions:

❑ Better control of dust
❑ Reduce animal dander
❑ Eliminate ways mold can grow
❑ Avoid plant allergens
❑ Other: _____

Become a psalmist like David, and write a poem thanking God for the privilege of caring for your own body:

_____

_____

_____

_____

_____

_____

_____

Chapter 4

Attacking Allergies Through Vitamins and Supplements

O ne night the psalmist David looked into a starry sky and thought about God the Creator and about himself, a marvelously unique creation. Listen to his beautiful words:

> When I look at the night sky and see the work of your fingers—the moon and the stars you have set in place—what are mortals that you should think of us, mere humans that you should care for us? For you made us only a little lower than God, and you crowned us with glory and honor. . . . O LORD, our Lord, the majesty of your name fills the earth!
>
> —PSALM 8:3–5, 9

David's heart was overwhelmed by God's creative power, and he was humbled by the touch of creative genius used in making mankind. I wonder, if we were a little more awed by God's creative handiwork in the masterpiece of who we are, would we be more attentive to the care of our bodies?

Through His marvelous creation, God has also supplied countless sources of nourishment. Vitamins and minerals are uniquely programmed by God to strengthen the many systems of our bodies.

Although you get them in some measure in the foods you eat, vitamins and minerals should be taken as supplements to strengthen your immune system and provide your body what it needs to fight the symptoms of allergies.

Food Allergies

If you are experiencing food allergies, your Bible Cure plan includes giving your body plenty of the following vitamins and supplements. These powerful nutrients will help to restore intestinal mucus back to health.

Glutamine. To heal the cells of the small intestines, I recommend two tablets, or 1,000 milligrams, of glutamine three times a day. Take them about thirty minutes before each meal.

I also recommend a combination product called Total Leaky Gut from Nutri-West. It contains glutamine, N-acetyl, glucosamine, DGL, slippery elm, lipoic acid, zinc and vitamins C and E. (DGL is a form of licorice that has had glycyrrhetinic acid removed, since glycyrrhetinic acid occasionally causes high blood pressure. You can find it at your local health food store.)

Bromelain is a digestive enzyme that will help you digest proteins. Bromelain comes from pineapples, and when it is absorbed, it has anti-inflammatory activity. Take 200 milligrams twice daily.

GLA, which is found in evening primrose oil, black currant oil or borage oil, is a fatty acid that the body converts to PGE_1, which has anti-inflammatory properties. The normal dose is approximately 300 milligrams a day; however, you may take up to 1,500 milligrams a day to suppress inflamation.

Taking the above nutrients daily will help your body to mend the integrity of the intestinal tract and will improve the way nutrition is absorbed into your bloodstream.

Environmental Allergies

If you sneeze, wheeze, cough and drain because of airborne allergens, the following list of vitamins and supplements will help you to strengthen the special needs of your immune system.

Vitamin C. I recommend 1,000 milligrams of buffered vitamin C, three times a day. High levels of buffered vitamin C in the body have an antihistamine effect. Vitamin C also helps to support the adrenals. In addition to strengthening the body against environmental allergens, vitamin C also helps the body fight withdrawal symptoms and reactions caused by eating foods you are allergic to.

Bioflavonoids are also effective against allergy symptoms. They are potent anti-inflammatories and are found in the white pith of citrus fruits and other foods containing vitamin C. Bioflavonoids boost the immune system and help limit histamine reactions. You can find them in vitamin and mineral supplements such as vitamin C with bioflavonoids.

> *Give all your worries and cares to God, for he cares about what happens to you.*
> —1 PETER 5:7

Quercetin is a bioflavonoid that reduces

histamine levels. Take quercetin in a dose of 500 milligrams three times a day, along with buffered vitamin C in a dose of 1,000 milligrams three times a day, to relieve allergy symptoms. Quercetin is also found in yellow and red onions.

Grape seed extract is another bioflavonoid that taken with vitamin C helps to suppress allergic reactions. I recommend a dose between 100 milligrams and 300 milligrams a day.

Pantothenic acid, or vitamin B_5, helps support both the adrenals and thymus gland, which will in turn minimize allergic responses. Take a dose of 300 to 500 milligrams per day.

Omega 3 fatty acid is fish oil. A dose of approximately two 1,000-milligram capsules taken at each meal may help protect against allergic attacks.

Stingy nettles have leaves that cause small protrusions that burn the skin when you touch them. These stingy leaves have an anti-inflammatory effect upon the body, especially when ingested together with vitamin C, and will reduce allergy symptoms. A normal dose is 200 to 300 milligrams of nettle capsules three times a day during allergy season.

As you are faithful to take these vitamins and supplements, you will strengthen your immune system and help your body fight off allergy symptoms to any environmental toxins you may encounter.

Conclusion

Your Creator has provided everything you need to strengthen, support and sustain you. He has graced the earth with vitamins and herbs to bless mankind. The Word of God says, "He causeth the grass to grow for the cattle, and herb for the service of man: that he may bring forth food out of the earth" (Ps. 104:14, KJV).

Remember that God has provided these natural substances to help you walk in divine health. As you pray, read scriptures, avoid toxins, eat right and take your vitamins and supplements, you will discover that your body begins to build a new strength against allergy symptoms that have made you miserable all of your life. Begin developing an allergy-free lifestyle today that will better enable you to worship and serve your Creator.

> *Don't be impressed with your own wisdom. Instead, fear the LORD and turn your back on evil. Then you will gain renewed health and vitality.*
> —PROVERBS 3:7–8

A BIBLE CURE PRAYER
FOR YOU

Father God, You have created so many wonderful substances to help my body stay healthy and fight off allergies. Help me remember each day to take the supplements I need for continued strength. Give me wisdom to avoid toxins in my environment and food. Make me a vessel dedicated to Your service. Amen.

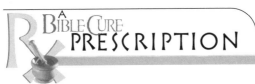

A BIBLE CURE PRESCRIPTION

Check the supplements you need to take to improve your intestinal digestion:

- ❏ Glutamine
- ❏ Bromelain
- ❏ GLA

Check the vitamins and supplements you plan to take to help you overcome your allergies:

- ❏ Vitamin C
- ❏ Quercetin
- ❏ Grape seed extract
- ❏ Pantothenic acid
- ❏ Omega 3 fatty acid
- ❏ Stingy nettles

Chapter 5

Arriving at Victory
Through the Power of Faith

Most doctors work hard at being good physicians. But there is only one Great Physician who is able to heal every disease. His name is Jesus Christ. By now I'm sure you realize that this Bible Cure involves looking to the Divine Healer who loves you dearly and has the power to make you well.

The Bible promises healing and health through faith and prayer to those who look to God and believe. The Word of God says, "Are any among you sick? They should call for the elders of the church and have them pray over them, anointing them with oil in the name of the Lord. And their prayer offered in faith will heal the sick, and the Lord will make them well" (James 5:14).

The power of faith and prayer are two of the most powerful forces in the universe. By faith and prayer any common person can touch the supernatural God. Have you considered asking someone to pray with you for your health? Perhaps you don't know an individual who can lead you in the prayer of faith for healing. That doesn't matter. You can bow your head right now and pray a prayer with me this very minute.

A BIBLE CURE PRAYER FOR YOU

Dear Jesus Christ, I thank You that You are the Great Physician who has the power to heal my body and make me completely well. I ask You to touch my body with Your mighty healing anointing right now. I believe that You died to save me and that You suffered on a cross to deliver me from my sufferings. I thank You for Your great love for me and Your mighty power. In Jesus' name, amen.

Isaiah 53:5 speaks of Jesus' death on the cross when it says, "But he was wounded and crushed for our sins. He was beaten that we might have peace. He was whipped, and we were healed!"

You see, Jesus Christ took your place of pain when He was beaten; He exchanged your penalty for sin when He was crucified. He actually traded places with you so that you could be healed. Now, I realize that this may be a little difficult to understand. God's ways are beyond our own. (See Isaiah 55:8.) But even if we cannot fully understand them, we can still choose to believe.

I have personally witnessed God's healing power in the lives of many individuals around the world, and I have experienced God's healing touch in my own body as well. That same healing power is available to you, too! It just takes a little faith.

A Word About Faith

So many people think that faith is a great, emotional power that some have and others don't. Nothing could be further from the truth. Faith is nothing more than a simple choice to take God at His Word. Faith simply chooses to believe God, even when circumstances, feelings and medical facts seem to contradict.

Here is another powerful truth about faith: Faith holds on. It doesn't give up or let go. I love the passage in the Bible about a woman who knocked at the door of a judge. When he didn't seem to hear, she kept knocking and she kept asking. Finally the judge got out of bed and gave her what she wanted. (See Luke 18:2–5.) The Bible says that Jesus told this parable to show how we should keep praying and not give up.

The Bible tells us that nothing is impossible if we have faith: "I assure you, even if you had faith as small as a mustard seed you could say to this mountain, 'Move from here to there,' and it would move. Nothing would be impossible" (Matt. 17:20).

I encourage you to choose to have faith, even if you are facing a mountain of allergy symptoms that you have battled all of your life. Be like the

> *O LORD my God, I cried out to you for help, and you restored my health.*
> —PSALM 30:2

woman and the judge—keep praying until you get your answer.

In addition, take the Bible Cure steps outlined in this booklet to strengthen your body, and prepare to feel better than you've ever felt!

A BIBLE CURE PRAYER
FOR YOU

I pray that God motivates you by His Spirit to apply all that you have learned. May you avoid all toxins and pollutants in your environment in your daily walk. May you never harm your body by breathing in smoke or other substances that can weaken your immune system and cause allergies. May God's healing work sustain and uplift you as you enjoy divine health and live life allergy free. Amen.

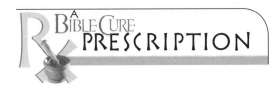

Describe how prayer and faith help to strengthen you spiritually to fight your allergies.

_____

_____

_____

_____

_____

_____

If you do not receive an immediate answer to prayer, what do you plan to do?

_____

_____

_____

_____

_____

_____

Memorize the following verses:

> He spoke, and they were healed—snatched from the door of death.
>
> —Psalm 107:20

> I will give you back your health and heal your wounds, says the Lord.
>
> —Jeremiah 30:17

Begin Your Allergy-Free Future Today!

Y ou now have a plan to live allergy free. It begins with understanding what is causing allergic reactions in your life. You may have discovered that certain toxins in your environment are prompting your allergic symptoms. You may be breathing in certain substances that your body reacts to. Or you may be eating and ingesting certain foods or chemicals that adversely affect your body.

Your knowledge is a gift from God to help you overcome allergies and live allergy free. God intends for you to live life abundantly in every respect. (See John 10:10.) You can live abundantly only if you have a healthy immune system that can resist all attacks from allergens. Through Scripture, prayer, good nutrition, eliminating toxins and allergens and taking the right supplements and vitamins, you can win a personal victory over allergies!

The best days of your life are ahead of you, free from sneezing, wheezing, watery eyes and other painful symptoms of allergies. By faith I believe that you will walk in divine health as you apply the wisdom and knowledge you have gained in this booklet.

—DON COLBERT, M.D.

Appendix

Dr. Colbert's Elimination Diet and Journal for Food Allergies

To determine what foods you are allergic to, you must first cleanse or detoxify your body from all the potential food allergens that you may now be eating. To do this, you will need to follow one of the following options (before beginning this elimination diet, consult with a nutritional doctor):

Option 1: Fast from all foods except water and Ultraclear or UltraInflamX (available from a nutritional doctor) for four days. It usually takes four to five days to clear out any food allergens from your system. If you cannot fast and take UltraInflamX or Ultraclear, then try option 2.

Option 2: Eliminate all foods from your diet except water, rice protein concentrate that can be used in a shake (obtain from a health food store),

71

a salad with dark green romaine lettuce, extra-virgin olive oil and lemon juice. Do not have any other additives to your lettuce. You may also have lamb, rice, chicken, broccoli, cabbage and apples. Eat this for four to five days.

Journal for a
Seven-Day Elimination Diet

Instructions:

Keep a journal of what you are eating and how much water you are drinking. Drink as many ounces of water as would equal to one-half your body weight. For example, if you weigh 150 pounds, then try to drink at least 75 ounces of water daily. Water is essential for flushing all the allergens and toxins from your system.

BIBLE CURE

Foods You Have Eaten	Time Eaten
_____	_____
_____	_____
_____	_____
_____	_____
_____	_____
_____	_____
_____	_____
_____	_____

How much water did you drink?

_____

BIBLE CURE

JOURNAL
DAY 2

Foods You Have Eaten	Time Eaten

How much water did you drink?

_____

BIBLE CURE

Foods You Have Eaten	Time Eaten

How much water did you drink?

_____

BIBLE CURE

Foods You Have Eaten	Time Eaten

How much water did you drink?

_____

Day 5

Instructions: Now that your body is cleansed, you can introduce the first set of foods that often create allergy symptoms in other people. You may discover that you develop some of the food allergy symptoms we mentioned on pages 12–14 within forty-eight hours. Take your pulse right before eating these potential allergens and immediately after eating them. If your pulse rate increases ten or more beats a minute, it is highly likely that you are allergic to this group of foods. You must take your pulse for a full minute.

The first set of potential allergens are eggs and products that contain eggs. Drink a shake of rice protein concentrate, eat a salad with extra-virgin olive oil and lemon juice, drink water and eat the other safe foods, but add eggs for one day. Follow the cleansing option you have chosen for two to three days to see if allergic symptoms occur. If you have an allergic reaction to eggs, then you have identified at least this one food allergen.

BIBLE CURE

Foods You Have Eaten	Time Eaten

How much water did you drink?

_____

Pulse rate for 1 minute
before eating eggs____

Pulse rate for 1 minute
immediately after eating eggs ____

BIBLE CURE

Foods You Have Eaten	Time Eaten
_____	_____
_____	_____
_____	_____
_____	_____
_____	_____
_____	_____
_____	_____
_____	_____

How much water did you drink?

_____

If you did not get an allergic reaction to eggs on the first day you tried them, you need to continue to watch for them through day 7 to be certain your body is not going to react to this allergen.

BIBLE CURE

Foods You Have Eaten	Time Eaten

How much water did you drink?

Instructions:

If you did not have an allergic reaction to eggs, then try the next potential allergen. Proceed through the two- to three-day testing cycle with each of the following food groups.

When you test the next potential food group allergen for a day, follow the day of eating the potential allergen food group with two to three days of observing and cleansing. Proceed through each food group until you have identified your food allergies.

Keep a journal like the one on the previous pages and simply substitute one of the following food groups for eggs. These are the food groups to test for potential allergic reactions.

Milk products: Butter, buttermilk, cheese, cottage cheese, cow's milk, cream cheese, goat's milk, ice cream, margarine, milk shakes, sour cream, yogurt

Wheat products: Bread, pasta, crackers, cereal, any foods made with wheat

Corn products: Check food labels for corn syrup, corn flour, grits, all foods made with corn-meal

Soy products: Soy flour, soy milk, tempeh, texturized soy protein, tofu

Other foods: I have also seen a number of food allergens to these foods that you may wish to test—peanuts, tomatoes, berries, sugar, chocolate, caffeine, etc.

Some people will discover that they have fixed food allergies to certain foods, which means that these foods will always produce allergic symptoms. Other people will have cyclic food allergies, which means if they eat the same foods every day, they will then develop allergic symptoms. I therefore recommend that patients eat a wide variety of foods and that they rotate foods over a four-day period. In other words, if you do not have a fixed allergy to eggs or milk products, but have a cyclic allergy to both, you can eat eggs and milk products on Monday. But then you will need to wait until Friday, which is four days, before you eat them again. By rotating these foods every four days, you are less likely to experience allergic symptoms.

Notes

PREFACE
YOU *WILL* FEEL BETTER!

1. "New Survey Reveals Allergies Nearly Twice As Common As Believed—Afflicting More Than One-Third of Americans," American College of Allergy, Asthma, and Immunology (ACAAI) 7/29/99 news release on www.allergy.mcg.edu.

CHAPTER 1
ALL ABOUT ALLERGIES

1. Adapted from the American College of Allergy, Asthma and Immunology, www.allergy.edu/quiz.
2. "About Food Allergies," The American College of Allergy, Asthma and Immunology, www.allergy.mcg.edu/ Advice/foods.

CHAPTER 2
ATTACKING ALLERGIES THROUGH NUTRITION

1. H. Leight Steward, et. al., *Sugar Busters* (New York: Ballantine Books, n.d.), 19.

CHAPTER 3
ATTACKING ALLERGIES THROUGH ENVIRONMENT

1. "Increase in Asthmas Associated with Indoor Allergens and Inactivity" 11/8/96 news release of the American College of Allergy, Asthma and Immunology, www. allergy.mcg.edu/news/indoor.

Don Colbert, M.D., was born in Tupelo, Mississippi. He attended Oral Roberts School of Medicine in Tulsa, Oklahoma, where he received a bachelor of science degree in biology in addition to his degree in medicine. Dr. Colbert completed his internship and residency with Florida Hospital in Orlando, Florida.

If you would like more
information about natural and
divine healing, or information about
Divine Health Nutritional Products®
you may contact
Dr. Colbert at:

DR. DON COLBERT

1908 Boothe Circle
Longwood, FL 32750
Telephone: 407-331-7007

Dr. Colbert's Web site is
www.drcolbert.com.

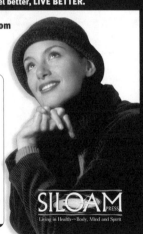

Pick up these other health-related
books from Siloam Press:

Walking in Divine Health

BY DON COLBERT, M.D.

You Are Not What You Weigh

BY LISA BEVERE

The Bible Cure

BY REGINALD CHERRY, M.D.

Healthy Expectations

BY PAMELA SMITH

Fit for Excellence!

BY SHERI ROSE SHEPHERD

The Hope of Living Cancer Free

BY FRANCISCO CONTRERAS, M.D.

Ultimate Living!

BY DEE SIMMONS

*Train Up Your Children in
the Way They Should Eat*

BY SHARON BROER

Maximum Energy

BY TED BROER

Available at your local bookstore
or call 1-800-599-5750
or visit our Web site at www.creationhouse.com